Sildenafil Vi

MW00875799

The Best Sex Guide to Blue Men Sex, and Instant, Fast Acting, Long Lasting (Long Time) Erection for a Mind Blowing, Screaming Big-O Climax for Her

SILVA BARROS

Table of Contents

CHAPTER ONE

Starting

A medication that is given to men who suffer from erectile dysfunction (ED), sildenafil citrate, which is more commonly known by its brand name Viagra, is a medication that is also used to treat a variety of heart disorders. Sildenafil citrate is a medicine that is more commonly known by its brand name Viagra (for example, pneumonic blood vessel hypertension). One of the different brand names that are available for Viagra is called Revatio.

Viagra, which was initially developed to relieve the pressure that was being exerted on the circulatory system, is now most commonly used in the treatment of erectile dysfunction. The effects of Viagra have, during the course of the drug's existence, been shown to have a substantial and positive influence on the manner in which men describe the caliber of their sexual encounters.

When used as directed, it normally takes Viagra roughly a half an hour to begin exerting its effect after the medication has been consumed. However, the length of time it takes for Viagra to start working in your body and the amount of time its effects continue to be effective can be affected by a wide variety of factors. These factors can range from how long it takes for Viagra to start working in your body to how long its effects continue to be effective. The food that you eat, your general health, any other prescriptions that you are currently taking, any hidden health problems, and a great deal more are some of these aspects. However, there are a great deal more.

CHAPTER TWO

How Viagra Works

Impotence, also known as erectile dysfunction, is a condition that affects men that happens when the nerves in a man's penis are unable to deliver the appropriate signals to the brain. Because of this, the corpora cavernosa, which are two chamber-shaped sections of flexible material along the penis, are unable to receive the blood flow necessary to produce an erection. Medical professionals use the phrase "erectile dysfunction" to refer to the inability to keep an erection going.

Viagra makes it possible for blood to flow more efficiently into the parts of the penis that are involved for producing an erection. This makes it possible for the patient to achieve and maintain an erection. This is made possible due to the fact that it relaxes the walls of the veins, which is how it produces its effect and makes it feasible for this to happen. Viagra makes it much easier to get and maintain an erection going because it causes more blood to flow to the penis. This makes it much simpler to have an erection in the first place.

When taken in tablet form, Viagra could start having an effect anywhere from thirty minutes to an hour after it has been swallowed, depending on how much of the medication was consumed.

Viagra doesn't create an erection all alone. In spite of everything, you will need to make sure that you are feeling an incredible amount of excitement in order for it to take place. You have a better chance of experiencing the benefits of Viagra more quickly if you are able to keep your composure and stay relaxed when you are taking the medication prescribed to you.

Viagra is only able to help people who struggle to get or hold erections successfully (people who have erectile brokenness) stay in bed for longer. This is because Viagra works by improving blood flow to the penile tissue. The medical name for the condition in which a person is unable to develop or maintain an erection correctly is referred to as erectile brokenness. It does not in any manner heal an erection that has been harmed. In the event that this occurs, you will be need to look for a different form of treatment in order to address your condition.

Viagra is effective for an average of between two and three hours before it begins to lose its properties, before its effects begin to wear off. This is before it begins to lose its effectiveness. It is also conceivable that it could last for up to five hours, or possibly even longer, depending on the measurements that are obtained, the digestive processes of the body, and any other external elements that may be present at the time. This would be the case if it lasted for longer than five hours. It could take the active ingredients in Viagra up to an hour to start working for men who have problems maintaining an erection after they have taken the medication. Before engaging in any sexual activity after taking Viagra, it is recommended that you wait at least four hours.

The effectiveness with which your body processes Viagra will determine the number of times you are able to acquire and keep an erection while it is still present in your system, as will the length of time that an erection may be maintained for.

Even though Viagra won't prevent your erection from getting weaker after you've reached your climax, you are free to continue having sexual encounters while the medicine is still working because it won't stop your erection from getting weaker in the first place. This is because Viagra won't stop your erection from getting weaker after you've reached your climax. Despite this, there is still a chance that you will require a break in between erections after you have hit your climax. This is because your blood supply may have been depleted.

Viagra, despite the fact that it is really helpful, is not going to be of any support with the following issues:

ϒ Premature discharge (coming too soon). Conduct

research to determine whether or not the treatment you are receiving is causing early discharge.

Υ Having the experience of being exhausted after having participated in sexual activity. Coffee consumption is one of the most effective ways to prevent feeling tired while engaging in sexual activity; however, improving your overall level of health is the single most beneficial method. Coffee consumption is one of the most effective ways to prevent feeling tired while engaging in sexual activity.

ϒ Insignificant sexual drives (low moxie). You can fight this by either getting treatment or making some adjustments to the way you currently conduct your life. Both are viable options.

It is possible that it will be many hours before all traces of Viagra are eliminated from the system. This is the case in the majority of cases. On the other hand, the amount of time it takes for the chemical to leave your system completely could range anywhere from five to six hours, and it all depends on how well you digest meals. The time it takes for the chemical to leave your system completely could range anywhere from five to six hours. In addition, the length of time it takes for the substance to be expelled from the body is taken into consideration when determining the severity of the actions to be taken. For instance, you might not notice the effects of a dose of 25 milligrams (mg) until after two or three hours, while it might take about three times as long for the effects of a dose of 100 mg to leave your system. This is because a higher dose causes a greater accumulation of the drug in your system. The reason for this is that taking a higher dose result in a greater buildup of the drug throughout your body.

If you feel as though Viagra is not working as quickly as you would like it to, you may want to try masturbation or foreplay in order to help raise arousal. This will allow you to get the most out of your experience with Viagra. You shouldn't take any more than the daily dose that was suggested by your primary care physician if it doesn't start functioning within the first half an hour. This is the most prudent thing to do in the situation. Because the blood that is held in the penis is not obtaining oxygen, this could lead to priapism, which is a painful erection that lasts for more than four hours and can cause damage to the tissue of the penis. Priapism can occur as a result of this. A person can protect themselves from developing priapism by avoiding foods that are rich in magnesium and potassium and by consuming a lot of water.

In the event that something similar takes place, you need to seek medical assistance as soon as it is feasible for you to do so.

CHAPTER THREE

The Dosage and Usage

If you are using Viagra to treat either erectile dysfunction or high blood pressure in the pulmonary arteries, the dosage that you take will be different from the dosage that you would take if you were using it to treat the other ailment (that is, pulmonary arterial hypertension).

Viagra is most typically seen in the form of blue pills shaped like valuable stones, and its dosages can range anywhere from 25 milligrams to 100 milligrams. The pill's design is what gives Viagra its trademark name. The medical condition known as erectile dysfunction can be treated with Viagra. It is necessary to take just one pill throughout the course of twenty-four hours, and you should take it anywhere from a half hour to an hour before indulging in sexual activity.

Viagra (Revatio), which is one of the drugs that can be used to treat aspiratory blood vessel hypertension, is available in the form of white, film-coated, spherical pills. Each time, you should take one tablet that is 20 milligrams, and you should take those tablets once every three hours.

It is not a laughing matter that it is possible to take too much of the drug Viagra. In the event that you have reason to believe that you may have consumed more than the amount that is recommended, you should get in touch with a qualified medical expert or the poison control center that serves your region as soon as possible.

The following is a list of potential adverse effects that could be the result of taking an excessive amount of a substance:

- ϒ Vomiting
- ϒ Diarrhea
- ϒ Blindness

- ϒ Eyesight that has been twisted and warped, as well as vision that has been disfigured and mutilated
- ϒ Neuropathy of the optic nerve (harm to the optic nerve)
- ϒ Priapism that lasts for a considerable amount of time and is not stopped.
- ϒ Papilledema (growing in the optic nerve)
- ϒ Tachycardia (that is expanded pulse)
- ϒ Rhabdomyolysis (separate of muscles)

In spite of the fact that it does not happen very frequently, there is always a possibility of passing away.

Before beginning treatment for erectile dysfunction with Viagra or any other medication that is analogous to it, you are required to discuss the matter at length with your primary care physician.

Viagra has the potential to have an adverse interaction with a variety of different drugs that are prescribed for the treatment of cardiac conditions. Nitroglycerin and a variety of other nitrates are among the drugs that are included in this category. Because of the combination between these two factors, it's possible that your blood pressure will decrease dramatically.

CHAPTER FOUR

Factors Effecting Viagra

There are a number of factors that, in addition to Viagra's dosage and length of use, can influence both its efficacy and how long it continues to work for an individual.

Diet

Before using Viagra, a meal that is either very rich or very heavy in fat will prevent the medicine from being absorbed as quickly or as well as it otherwise would be. It will be more challenging to achieve and maintain an erection as a result of this. On the other hand, if you use it in conjunction with your dinner, it can help to make it last for a longer period of time, which is a benefit that you can take advantage of. If the medication is taken on an empty stomach first thing in the morning, it will be able to begin exerting its positive effects on the body much more swiftly.

Liquor

Consuming alcohol reduces the volume of blood that flows to the penis, which makes it more difficult to obtain and maintain an erection once one has been established. If you take Viagra and consume a significant amount of alcohol at the same time, your risk of having undesirable side effects may increase, and you may discover that you are unable to achieve or maintain an erection.

Age

In most cases, as time goes on, a senior citizen's digestive tract loosens up and becomes less tense. It's possible that the effects will continue to have an effect on men who are at least 65 years old for another two or three years after they've experienced them.

Dosage

After you take Viagra, the amount of the drug that will stay in your system is directly proportional to the dosage that you initially took of the drug. The majority of the time, taking a higher dosage will result in superior outcomes, and those outcomes will be maintained for a lengthier amount of time. Get in touch with your primary care physician so that he or she can recommend the appropriate amount for you; it isn't always recommended to take a greater quantity because it could not be safe to do so. Your primary care physician can recommend the appropriate dose for you.

Meds

Clarithromycin (Biaxin), erythromycin (Ery-Tab), and

ciprofloxacin (Cipro), amongst other antibacterial medications, have the potential to influence both the strength of Viagra as well as the amount of time it takes for the drug to take action. Make an appointment with your primary care physician to see whether or not you are at risk for any interactions between the medications you take by scheduling an appointment today.

Mental State

Discomfort, anxiety, tension, or wretchedness can all affect how your body reacts when it is stimulated sexually, and this can have an effect on how your body responds. If you are suffering any of these situations, it is possible that the effects of Viagra will not be as strong or that the drug will not last as long. Before beginning to take Viagra, you should consult your physician if you are suffering any of these problems.

Wellbeing

The conditions that are now taking place in your body have an effect not only on the amount of time that Viagra continues to work for you but also on how well it performs its intended function. Diabetes, conditions that affect the sensory system like multiple sclerosis (MS), and heart conditions like atherosclerosis (fat buildup in the veins) are some examples of conditions that can reduce the effectiveness of Viagra and cause it to not last as long. Other conditions that can have this effect include conditions that affect the nervous system like multiple sclerosis (MS). Conditions that have an impact on the neurological system, such as lupus and lupus nephritis, are examples of other diseases that can have this kind of consequence. When compared to people who do not have these illnesses, those who suffer from specific hepatic or renal diseases may find that the effects of Viagra last for a significantly longer period of time than those who do not have these conditions. This is due to the fact that Viagra needs to be disassembled into its component parts.

CHAPTER FIVE

Viagra and Its Safety

Taking Viagra shouldn't put you at risk for any severe adverse effects as long as you follow the instructions that come with the medication. Despite this, there is a wide range of potentially harmful effects on a person's body if they consume it.

As shown by the results of preliminary clinical studies, the following is a list of the adverse responses to Viagra that have been recorded by the majority of individuals who have used the medication:

- ϒ A disorder that results in a diminished ability to see
- ϒ Indigestion
- ϒ Nasal blockage
- ϒ Photophobia (affectability to light)
- ϒ Headaches

On the other hand, responses could include any combination of the following:

- ϒ Sudden hearing misfortune
- ϒ Rhythm problems that originate in the lower chambers of the heart (the ventricles).
- ϒ An assault on the center of the chest

- ϒ A rise in the amount of pressure that is already present within the eye due to a buildup of fluid.
- ϒ Priapism (difficult dependable erection). This incidence is relatively uncommon.

A couple of our customers have stated to us that, under extremely exceptional conditions, they have had the experience of having cyanopsia. Cyanopsia is a form of colorblindness that causes a person to see everything as having a bluish tone. People with this form of colorblindness have cyanopsia.

The use of Viagra has also been linked, albeit in extremely isolated instances, to a kind of optic neuropathy known as nonarthritic foremost ischemic optic neuropathy. This form of optic neuropathy is characterized by progressive vision loss (that is harm to the optic nerve).

It has been suggested that regular use of Viagra can gradually reduce the amount of blood that travels to the optic nerve, which has been linked to an unexpected loss of eyesight. These claims have been made based on anecdotal evidence. In spite of this, the condition is highly rare, and research has shown that it is more prevalent in individuals who have diabetes, high cholesterol, a history of eye problems, cardiovascular illness, or high blood pressure.

People who are currently coping with HIV and taking protease inhibitors should discuss the possibility of using Viagra with their primary care physician as soon as possible. This is due to the fact that protease inhibitors not only increase the probability of reactions but also the intensity of those events. If a person is in this situation, they should not take more than 25 milligrams of Viagra at one time or over the course of forty-eight hours combined.

In a similar vein, individuals who take alpha-blockers should make sure that they take Viagra at least four hours before or after taking their alpha-blockers in order to assist in preventing a pulse rate that is dangerously low. This will help prevent an individual from experiencing a cardiac arrest. This is done in the hope that it will aid in the prevention of a cardiac arrest from taking place.

CHAPTER SIX

Who to Avoid Viagra

Due to the high cost of Viagra, it is not a treatment option that can be made available to everyone. This product is geared toward adult males who are at least 18 years old and are of the gender male. Consumption by females or children is absolutely forbidden in any and all circumstances. This may not be done by either of the two groups.

People who are attending a gathering are not permitted to use Viagra, or they must first discuss the matter with their primary care physician:

- ϒ Patients who are experiencing problems with either their hearts or their livers
- ϒ Patients who have been hospitalized for an extended period of time and have a history of having a stroke or cardiovascular failure
- ϒ Patients who have been told that they have renal disease
- ϒ Patients that suffer from a degenerative condition of the retina that has been passed down through their families (that is individuals with uncommon acquired eye infection)

ϒ Those who suffer from hypotension, often known as low blood pressure (low circulatory strain)

ϒ Individuals who are medicated with nitrates for the treatment of chest discomfort and who are consequently receiving nitric oxide contributors, nitrates, and natural nitrites. Individuals who are taking nitrates as a preventative measure against chest discomfort.

ϒ Patients who have previously shown an unfavorably susceptible reaction to Viagra or to one of the other drugs are not suitable for this treatment. Patients who have shown an unfavorably susceptible reaction to Viagra or to one of the other treatments.

٢ If a man has been cautioned about the increased risk of cardiovascular disease, it is recommended that he refrain from engaging in sexual activity as a kind of self-preservation.

Made in United States
Troutdale, OR
12/10/2023

15601438R10024